DIANE MOTISE

Dining Out Healthy Hacks

The Ultimate Guide to Making Healthy Choices While Eating Out Anytime, Anywhere, to Help Manage Your Weight and Health While Dieting, Traveling, or Just Meeting Friends

This book was professionally typeset on Reedsy.
Find out more at reedsy.com

Contents

Introduction

This book is a simple, step-by-step guide that will help anyone who dines out make the healthiest choices possible from virtually any restaurant, fast food drive-thru, or even a local grocery store deli, without giving up the pleasure of eating tasty food. You'll find super helpful tips on how to eat healthy at any meal - breakfast, lunch or dinner, anytime, anywhere.

My name is Diane Motise and I am a Registered Dietitian Nutritionist. I have been teaching weight loss and healthy lifestyle classes since 2001 and have had the privilege of helping hundreds of people of all ages lose weight and get healthier. This is my life's passion and it is so incredibly rewarding for me to be able to help others regain their health, their energy, and their zest for life!

One of the biggest challenges I hear over and over again from people everywhere is that it's so hard to stay on track with eating healthy and avoiding weight gain when they eat out - and we ALL eat out. It's a way of life for most of us. And just like you, I've struggled myself with the balancing act of enjoying dining out while staying true to my health goals. Dining out is one of my favorite pastimes. I am just as tempted as the next person by a juicy, charbroiled rib eye, a fresh baked, brick oven pizza covered in pepperoni and gooey mozzarella cheese, or a seven layer, dark chocolate ganache-filled cake. This book was borne out of my own experiences - successful and not so successful - in learning how to navigate the tricky landscape of restaurant menus, and finding my way to managing my weight and health and still getting to enjoy my food when I eat out. As someone who is passionate about both good food and good health, I wanted to create a resource that is very easy to read with very clear and simple steps to follow that can help anyone become a skilled connoisseur of eating out healthily at any restaurant - anytime, anywhere.

As you just read, I used the word "skilled". Healthy dining rarely occurs with will power alone. Will power is fleeting, and eventually, if put to the test enough times, it wanes... and we eventually give in to our temptations. It takes "skill power" - practicing various techniques and strategies over and over again until we become an expert at healthy dining. It's like learning a new language. We start with a few words and phrases, test them out, and when we use them enough we develop more confidence and begin trying more and more until we become fluent in our new way of speaking - only here we become fluent in a new way of eating - for health. That is the main goal of this book - to provide you with the coaching and the skills that will help you become a master at eating out AND maintaining a healthy body.

Why This Book?

Dining Out Healthy Hacks is a book that can help virtually everyone dine healthier. Whether you're a busy professional with little time to cook, a frequent traveler looking for healthy options on the road, a family of five in need of something quick and nutritious between soccer games and scout meetings, or someone who just enjoys hanging with friends and sharing the experience of eating good food together, this book is for you. The idea is simple: you don't have to sacrifice taste or the joy of eating out to stay on track with your health goals.

In today's fast-paced world, dining out has become more than just an occasional treat—it's a way of life. From quick stops at fast food joints to lavish dinners at gourmet restaurants, eating out is woven into the fabric of our social and professional lives. However, along with the convenience of dining out comes the challenge of making healthier choices amidst menus often laden with high-calorie, high-fat, and high-sugar options that inevitably put some major dents in our health plans. This book aims to empower you with the knowledge and strategies to make better choices, ensuring that you can enjoy your meals without guilt or compromise.

What Will Be Covered?

Throughout this book, you will find practical, step-by-step guidance on how to navigate any dining scenario. Here's a snapshot of what we'll cover:

1. **Deciding Where to Eat:** Learn how to choose restaurants that offer healthier options, understand the importance of menu research, and discover the benefits of planning ahead.

2. **Navigating the Menu:** Master the art of decoding menu descriptions, identifying healthier preparation methods, and asking the right questions to your server.

3. **Choosing a Balanced, Healthy Meal:** Understand the principles of a balanced diet and how to apply them to your restaurant choices, including tips on portion control and making smart substitutions.

4. **Calories Count and Estimating is Easy**: Get tips on estimating calorie counts, using available nutritional information, and making lower-calorie swaps without sacrificing taste.

5. **Think Mediterranean Diet and You'll Cover the Bases for Healthy**

Eating: It's actually not just a diet - it's a way of life. Living a Mediterranean lifestyle involves more than just following a specific diet - it's about embracing a holistic approach to health and well-being. Learn the simple how-to's of the number-one-ranked healthiest diet in the world.

6. **Additional Tips for Keeping Meals Healthy and Portion Controlled:** Learn advanced strategies for managing portions, avoiding common pitfalls, and maintaining your health goals even in the most challenging dining situations.

Each chapter is designed to provide you with actionable tips and insights that you can apply immediately. Whether you're dining at a fast food drive-thru, a local grocery store deli, or a Michelin Star restaurant, these hacks will help you make healthier choices effortlessly.

How Will This Benefit You?

By the end of this book, you will have a crystal clear understanding of how to make healthier choices while dining out. You will feel confident and empowered to enjoy your meals, knowing that you are making decisions that align with your health and weight goals. The strategies and tips provided in this guide will not only help you stay on track but also enhance your overall dining experience, allowing you to savor each meal without the worry of compromising your health.

Now that we've set the stage for your journey to healthier dining out, it's time to dive into the specifics. In the next chapter, we'll start with the very first step: deciding where to eat. You'll learn how to identify restaurants that cater to healthier choices and how to make informed decisions before you even step out the door. Get ready to embark on a journey that will transform the way you approach dining out, making it a joyous and health-conscious experience.

Welcome to **Dining Out Healthy Hacks**, your ultimate guide to making smart, healthy choices while enjoying the pleasure of eating out no matter where you go.

2

Deciding Where to Eat

Choosing where to eat is the first step in ensuring a healthy dining experience. With a little planning and awareness, you can find a restaurant that not only satisfies your taste buds but also aligns with your health goals, budget, and location. In this chapter, we'll explore how to make informed decisions about where to eat, covering everything from identifying restaurants that serve your preferred type of food to assessing their healthiness, pricing, and proximity.

Finding a Place to Eat That Serves the Type of Food You Want

The first consideration when deciding where to eat is your craving or preference for a particular type of food. Whether you're in the mood for Italian, Japanese, Mexican, or a simple sandwich, identifying your culinary desire can help narrow down your options. Here are some tips to guide you:

1. **Identify Your Cravings:** Think about what you're in the mood for. Are you craving a hearty meal, something light, or perhaps a specific cuisine?

2. **Use Apps and Websites:** Take advantage of the resourceful apps like Yelp, Zomato, or OpenTable, which allow you to filter options based on cuisine type, ratings, and customer reviews, or use your favorite search engine like Google or Safari to look for restaurants near you. These platforms often have detailed descriptions and ample photos from recent visitors that can help you make a decision.

3. **Ask for Recommendations:** Don't hesitate to ask friends, family, or colleagues for their favorite spots, and often the popular neighborhood apps like Nextdoor can provide great suggestions. Personal recommendations can often lead you to hidden gems that you might not find otherwise. If you are out of town, ask the concierge at your hotel or employee of any local establishment for recommendations based on their own experiences or customer feedback.

4. **Social Media:** Check social media platforms like Instagram or Facebook for restaurant reviews and food photos. Many restaurants post their daily specials and menus, which can help you decide if they have what you're craving.

How to Determine if a Restaurant Has Healthy Food Options

Once you've narrowed down the type of food you want, the next step is to ensure the restaurant offers healthy options. Here's how to evaluate whether a restaurant aligns with your health goals:

1. **Research Menus Online:** Many restaurants post their menus online. Look for sections dedicated to healthier choices, such as "lighter fare", "heart-healthy", or "vegetarian/vegan options".

2. **Check for Nutritional Information:** Some restaurants, especially chains, provide nutritional information on their websites or in-store. This can help you gauge the calorie, fat, and sodium content of different dishes.

3. **Look for Healthy Cooking Methods:** Pay attention to how food

is prepared. Opt for places that offer grilled, baked, steamed, or roasted dishes rather than fried or creamy options.

4. **Read Reviews and Ratings:** Customer reviews on platforms like Yelp or TripAdvisor can provide insights into the healthiness of the food. Look for mentions of fresh ingredients, portion sizes, and the availability of healthy options.

5. **Ask the Restaurant:** Don't be afraid to call ahead or ask the staff about their healthy menu options. Restaurants that prioritize customer health will be happy to provide this information.

How to See Pricing of Menu Options at Local Restaurants

Budget is an important factor when deciding where to eat. Here's how to assess the pricing of menu options:

1. **Online Menus:** Check the restaurant's website or food delivery apps like UberEats, DoorDash, or GrubHub, which often list detailed menus with prices.

2. **Review Sites:** Websites like Yelp, Zomato, or TripAdvisor typically include a price range ($, $$, $$$, $$$$) based on the average cost per person, which can give you a quick idea of the restaurant's affordability. Here's a general breakdown of what each dollar sign typically means:

3. $: Inexpensive. Meals are usually under $10 per person.

4. $$: Moderately priced. Meals range from $10 to $25 per person.

5. $$$: Expensive. Meals range from $25 to $50 per person.

6. $$$$: Very Expensive. Meals tend to be over $50 per person.

7. **Ask for a Menu:** If you're passing by a restaurant, you can often ask for a takeout menu or see if they have one displayed outside. This can give you a good sense of pricing before you decide to dine in.

8. **Special Offers and Discounts:** Look for special deals, happy hour

menus, or discounts. Many restaurants offer daily specials or promotions that can make dining out more affordable.

Proximity of the Restaurants or Food Establishments to Your Location

Convenience is key, especially when you're hungry. Here's how to find restaurants close to your location:

1. **Map Applications:** Use Google Maps or Apple Maps to search for nearby restaurants. These apps can provide distance, travel time, and directions.
2. **Restaurant Finder Apps:** Apps like Yelp, Zomato, TripAdvisor and OpenTable allow you to filter search results by distance, making it easy to find options close to you.
3. **Delivery and Takeout Services:** If you prefer to eat at home, services like UberEats, DoorDash, and GrubHub show which restaurants deliver to your location.
4. **Walk or Drive Around:** Sometimes the best way to find a new favorite spot is by exploring your surrounding area. Walk or drive around and note any interesting places you'd like to try.

Deciding where to eat involves a balance of taste preferences, health goals, budget, and convenience. By taking a proactive approach and utilizing available resources, you can find restaurants that meet all your criteria. In the next chapter, we'll dive deeper into how to navigate a menu to make the healthiest choices possible. Get ready to become a savvy diner who can enjoy eating out without compromising on health.

3

Navigating the Menu

O nce you've decided where to eat, the next step is mastering the menu to make healthy choices. Menus can be overwhelming with their numerous options, but with a little knowledge and strategy, you can navigate them effectively. This chapter will guide you through understanding menu offerings and recognizing both healthy and unhealthy indicators on menus, whether you're at a fast food spot, a restaurant, or a deli.

Getting Familiar with All That Is Offered on the Menu

Before diving into specifics, take a moment to familiarize yourself with the entire menu. Here's how to do it:

1. **Scan the Entire Menu:** Take a few minutes to read through the entire menu before making any decisions. This will help you understand the variety of options available and avoid missing out on potentially healthier choices that might be listed in less obvious sections.

2. **Pay Attention to Sections:** Menus are often divided into sections

such as appetizers, main dishes, sides, and desserts. Identify where healthier options might be located, like salads or grilled items.

3. **Look for Specialty Menus:** Some restaurants offer specialty menus for health-conscious customers, including gluten-free, vegetarian, vegan, or heart-healthy options. These can often be found on a separate page or at the back of the main menu.

4. **Ask Questions:** Don't hesitate to ask your server for recommendations or clarifications about menu items. They can often suggest healthier options or modifications.

Identify Words That Indicate the Food May Be a Healthy Option

Certain words on a menu can signal that a dish is likely to be healthier. Here's what to look for:

1. **Cooking Methods:** Terms like "grilled", "steamed", "baked", "broiled", "poached", or "roasted" often indicate healthier cooking methods that use less fat and retain more nutrients.

2. **Ingredient Keywords:** Look for dishes that highlight healthy ingredients like "fresh", "organic", "seasonal", "whole grain", "lean", "vegetable", or "fruit".

3. **Portion Indicators:** Words like "half portion", "small", or "appetizer size" can help you control portion sizes and reduce calorie intake.

4. **Customization Options:** Menus that mention "substitute", "on the side", or "no sauce" show that the restaurant is flexible and allows you to make healthier adjustments.

5. **Happy Hour:** These menus often contain smaller portions and as an added bonus are typically offered at reduced price.

Identify Words That Indicate the Food May Be Too High-Calorie and Unhealthy

Conversely, some menu terms can signal higher-calorie, less healthy options. These types of foods are often the ones we crave because of their indulgent and taste bud-stimulating ingredients, but these are detrimental to our weight and health goals. Here's what to watch out for and avoid whenever possible:

1. **Cooking Methods:** Words like "fried", "deep-fried", "crispy", "breaded", "battered", "melted", "sauteed", or "smothered" often mean the dish is cooked with a lot of oil or butter, adding extra calories and fat.

2. **Descriptive Words:** Be wary of dishes described as "creamy", "buttery", "cheesy", "sauced", "rich", or "loaded" which typically indicate high levels of fats, creams, and sugars.

3. **Portion Size Indicators:** Terms like "jumbo", "giant", "platter", or "combo" usually denote larger portion sizes that can lead to overeating.

4. **Sugar and Fat Alerts:** Words like "glazed", "candied", "syrup", or "caramelized" often signal added sugars, while "au gratin", "alfredo", "scalloped", "special sauce" or "with bacon" can indicate higher fat content.

5. **Avoid "All-You-Can-Eat" buffets, salad bars and "Bottomless Bowls or Plates":** They often contain high-calorie, high fat, high sodium, and low nutritional quality indulgent items that can tempt even the most dedicated health-driven diner to eat more than intended and sabotage anyone's weight and health goals.

By getting familiar with all that is offered on the menu and learning to recognize both healthy and unhealthy indicators, you can make informed choices that align with your health goals. In the next chapter, we'll delve deeper into how to build a balanced, healthy meal from these choices.

Get ready to take your dining out experience to the next level, making it both enjoyable and health-conscious.

4

Choosing a Balanced, Healthy Meal

Eating balanced, healthy meals is essential for maintaining good health, managing weight, and ensuring your body gets the nutrients it needs. If your ultimate goal is to develop and maintain a healthy body at a healthy weight, choosing foods that create a balanced, healthy meal is a must.This chapter will define what balanced, healthy eating is, why it's important, and how to use the MyPlate model to make informed meal choices. Additionally, we will provide tips on selecting meals with healthy proteins, starches, vegetables, fruits, and fats.

What Does It Mean to Eat Balanced and Healthy?

Balanced, healthy eating involves consuming a variety of foods in the right proportions to provide your body with essential nutrients. A balanced meal typically includes a mix of macronutrients (proteins, carbohydrates, and fats) and micronutrients (vitamins and minerals). Key elements of a balanced diet include:

1. **Variety:** Eating a wide range of foods to ensure you get different

14

nutrients.

2. Moderation: Controlling portion sizes and not overeating any particular food group.
3. **Nutrient Density:** Choosing foods that are rich in vitamins, minerals, and other nutrients but relatively low in calories.
4. **Eating the MyPlate way:** This is a very simple visual of how to include the most important components of a meal to make it a complete and nutritionally balanced meal.

Why Should We Eat Healthy?

Eating a healthy, balanced diet is crucial for several reasons:

1. **Physical Health:** Reduces the risk of chronic diseases such as heart disease, diabetes, and cancer.
2. **Weight Management:** Helps in maintaining a healthy weight or achieving weight loss.
3. **Energy Levels:** Provides the energy needed for daily activities and improves overall vitality.
4. **Mental Health:** Supports healthy brain function and emotional well-being.
5. **Longevity:** Contributes to a longer, healthier life.

What Is the MyPlate?

MyPlate is a visual guide created by the United States Department of Agriculture (USDA) to help individuals make healthier food choices. It provides a simple, easy-to-understand visual of what a balanced meal should look like. MyPlate is divided into five food groups:

1. **Vegetables:** Encourages including a variety of colorful vegetables, especially dark green, red, and orange vegetables, as well as legumes and at every meal.

2. **Fruits:** Emphasizes whole fruits rather than fruit juices.
3. **Grains:** At least half of your grains should be whole grains.
4. **Protein:** Includes lean meats, poultry, seafood, beans, peas, nuts, seeds, and soy products.
5. **Dairy:** Recommends low-fat or fat-free dairy products 2-3 servings per day.

Explain How to Eat Using the MyPlate

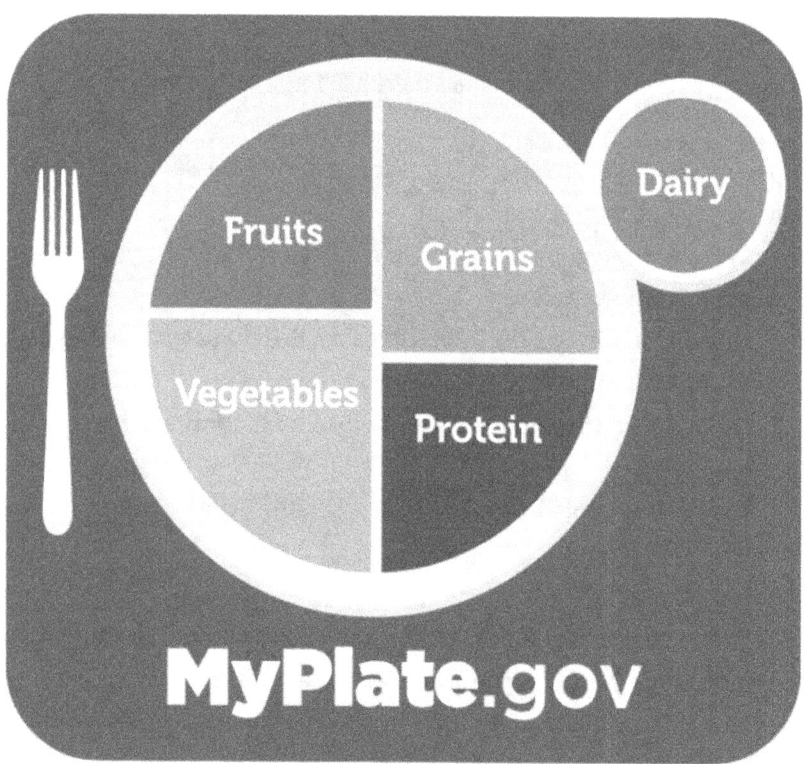

Using the MyPlate visual as a guide, here's how to create a balanced meal:

1. **Make Half Your Plate Vegetables and/or Fruits:** Aim to fill half of your plate or half the entire bulk of the meal with a mix of vegetables and/or fruits. They provide essential vitamins, minerals, fiber and are excellent sources of health promoting antioxidants and phytochemicals. They also provide volume which can help you feel fuller while eating smaller portions of the higher calorie carbohydrates and protein, and they can add eye-appealing color which can make a meal more appetizing.

2. **Make One Fourth Your Plate Grains or Starchy Vegetables:** Fill a quarter of your plate with wholesome grains or healthy starchy vegetables. They are rich in complex carbohydrates that provide vital energy to the brain, muscles, and heart which help them to function optimally. They also provide fiber, essential vitamins, minerals and phytonutrients that play a role in maintaining a healthy gut microbiome. These nutrients support overall health and can help prevent diseases like heart disease and cancer. Starches are a must at every meal, and for me as a dietitian, that is non-negotiable. The brain needs those healthy starchy carbs as its primary fuel source, and they give real satiety to the meal. Oftentimes when starches are left out of a meal the brain may start to speak loudly to you later in a way saying "hey, you forgot about me!" and sends out a craving to eat some carbs asap, which frequently can lead us to looking for something sweet or starchy like crackers, cookies or dessert. The brain is asking for glucose - its preferred fuel.

3. **Make One Fourth Your Plate Protein:** The remaining quarter should be protein. Including protein in your meals is crucial for several reasons. Protein helps you feel full longer, is essential for maintaining, building and repairing muscle tissue, is beneficial for bone health by helping maintain bone mass and reduce the risk of osteoporosis and fractures, and is vital for the repair and growth of virtually every cell in the body. Choose lean protein sources

such as chicken breast, ground turkey, fish or other seafood, beans, or tofu. Many restaurants offer vegetarian versions of burgers, chicken tenders, eggs, etc. which can be healthy options for most vegetarians or vegans.

4. **Include Dairy Daily:** Ideally, you'll want to add two to three servings of dairy daily as part of your meals or snacks such as a glass of low fat milk, cottage cheese, lower calorie cheese like feta, goat, mozzarella or parmesan, or a serving of low fat regular or Greek yogurt. If I were to ask you what's the main nutrient found in these dairy products that is vital for healthy bones and good heart health, what might you say? Yes, it's calcium. And these foods are also great sources of protein, vitamin D, phosphorus, magnesium and B12, all important for optimal health.

Ways to Add Healthy Vegetables and/or Fruits as Part of the Meal

Vegetables and fruits should be a significant part of your meal for their nutrient density and fiber content. If anyone asks me which food group is the most important one for overall health I will always say without hesitation - the Vegetable and Fruit Group. It contains so many of the illness-preventing, immune-boosting, and cancer-fighting nutrients that keep our bodies healthy. They are an absolute must if you want to create and maintain a healthy body for healthy longevity. Here's how to include them:

1. **Salads and Sides:** Opt for salads or vegetable sides. The more, the better. Choose dishes that feature a variety of colorful vegetables. If you don't see any on the menu, always ask the staff - they may have options available that may not have made it onto the menu.

2. **Vegetable-Rich Entrees:** Look for entrees that include a substantial amount of vegetables, such as stir-fries, vegetable soups, or casseroles.

3. **Fresh Fruit:** Add fresh fruit as a dessert or side. Fruit salads, fruit parfaits, or simply a piece of whole fruit can complement your meal and give you a healthy boost of nutrition.

4. Take a look at the vegetables and fruits that are served with other items on the menu. If you see something you'd like and it's not included with your selection, ask to substitute. If it's on the menu, it most likely can be served with your meal.

5. Feel free to add more than what is served with your meal anytime and anywhere! More is better in this case for optimal health.

Look for Meals That Contain Healthy Starches

Healthy starches are crucial for providing energy to the brain, heart and muscles, they contain gut-healthy fiber, and they provide other essential nutrients for optimal health. Look for:

1. **Whole Grains:** Choose whole grain options as often as possible such as brown rice, quinoa, whole wheat pastas and breads, bulgur, barley, whole grain dry cereals and oatmeal, corn or whole grain tortillas or wraps.

2. **Starchy Vegetables:** Include starchy vegetables like potatoes, sweet potatoes, corn, peas, butternut and acorn squash.

3. **Legumes:** Beans such as pinto, black and red, lentils, edamame, and peas are excellent sources of both protein and healthy starches.

4. No matter what, if whole grains or the above options are not available, it's always better to choose some kind of carb/starch, whole grain or not, than not including any.

Look for Meals That Contain Healthy Proteins

When selecting meals, aim for sources of lean protein that are lower in saturated fat and calories. Here are some tips:

1. **Lean Meats:** Choose options like chicken breast, turkey, lean cuts of red meat such as beef or pork tenderloin.
2. **Seafood:** Fish such as salmon, trout, tuna, halibut, tilapia, sole, flounder, and sardines are excellent choices as they are rich in omega-3 fatty acids and high in protein.
3. **Plant-Based Proteins:** Consider beans, lentils, chickpeas, tofu, tempeh, and edamame for vegetarian protein options.
4. **Eggs and Low-Fat Dairy:** Eggs are a versatile protein source and many dining establishments will offer egg whites or egg substitutes as a lower calorie option, and low-fat dairy products like Greek yogurt and cottage cheese can also contribute significantly to your protein intake.

Look for Healthy Fat Options AND Minimize the Amount of Fat Added to a Meal

While fats are necessary for a balanced diet, it's important to choose healthy fats and limit the amount. Here's how:

1. **Add Healthy Fats:** Opt for meals that include sources of healthy fats such as avocados, nuts, seeds, and olive oil.
2. **Avoid Unhealthy Fats:** Steer clear of foods high in saturated and trans fats. Avoid items that are deep-fried or heavily processed. The most common foods high in saturated fats are: ground beef/burgers, steaks, bacon, sausage, salami, pepperoni, cheese, bacon, butter and cream, ice cream, coconut oil. Saturated fats are linked to increased LDL (bad) cholesterol and increased risk of cardiovascular disease and should be limited to eating only once in a while and in small amounts. Trans fats are another health issue and are typically found in foods prepared with hydrogenated or partially hydrogenated oils so check labels and become familiar with these types of foods so you can avoid them as much as possible.

3. **SPECIAL NOTE:** I know… you're thinking "but those are all the typical foods I enjoy eating when I eat out!" That's the dilemma, and something you'll need to agree to change, even if it's little by little, if you are truly trying to make the changes necessary to create that healthy body you desire. It's about learning new behaviors and trying new things that will make life better for you health wise in the long run.

4. **Request Modifications:** Ask for dressings, sauces, and gravies on the side so you can control the amount. Request that your food be prepared with less oil or butter. All of these typically add fat calories quickly and can hinder our goals to maintain an appropriate calorie intake and trigger weight gain very quickly.

5. **Cooking Methods:** Choose dishes that are grilled, baked, steamed, or poached rather than fried or sautéed in large amounts of oil. And If the item you choose does not say "grilled, steamed, roasted or poached" ask if they can prepare it in any of those methods. It cannot hurt to ask, but can surely help with managing your calories and health. Anytime you can cut calories by selecting a healthier preparation of your food is a win for you.

6. **Understand the Importance of Fat Grams and Calories:** This is one of my most important coaching points. Paying attention to total fat grams and calories is vital for several reasons. Frequent excess calorie intake can lead to weight gain and often is associated with health issues like obesity, heart disease, and diabetes. Foods high in total fat grams can quickly push you over your fat intake limit for the day and drive up excess fat storage in your body. Fat grams, at 9 calories per gram, have more than double the calories of protein and carbohydrate grams, both of which contain 4 calories per gram. Similarly, high-fat diets, especially those rich in saturated and trans fats, can increase cholesterol levels and the risk of heart disease. By monitoring your fat intake as well as your total calorie

intake, you have a better chance of maintaining a balanced diet that supports your overall health and wellness goals. Lower the fat content whenever you can to help decrease the calorie content and minimize health risks associated with taking in too much fat.

Understanding balanced, healthy eating and using the MyPlate model can significantly improve the quality of your dining choices. By focusing on including healthy proteins, starches, vegetables, fruits, and fats, you can create meals that support your health goals while still being enjoyable. In the next chapter, we will discuss the importance of calories and how to count them effectively to stay on track with your health objectives. Get ready to become a pro at building nutritious and delicious meals no matter where you dine.

Restaurant Foods That Are Typically High in Fat

We just learned that it's essential to be aware of foods that are typically high in fats when dining out. Here are some common restaurant items that often contain high amounts of fats and are best to avoid or minimize how often you eat them. The list is not exhaustive, but it is a really great start to learning to identify these types of foods and to choosing to stay clear of them.

Fried Foods:

1. French Fries: Deep-fried and often cooked in oils high in trans fats.
2. Fried Chicken: Typically breaded and fried in oil, making it high in fat and calories.
3. Fried Fish or Seafood: Breaded and fried, similar to fried chicken.
4. Onion Rings: Deep-fried and often battered, contributing to high fat content.

Fast Food Items

1. Burgers: Especially those with multiple patties, cheese, bacon, and special sauces. I often like to use the following strategy to help shave calories off my meals. If the burger or sandwich or entire meal comes with multiple high fat, high calorie ingredients, I will allow myself to include one of the fatty ingredients that I really want to eat and leave out the others. Example - a burger comes with bacon, cheese, mayo and avocado. I might really want the cheese, so I'll ask to leave off the bacon, mayo and avocado. This can significantly reduce the calories of the meal up to several hundred calories, and I still get to feel like I've indulged some by adding the cheese.
2. Chicken Nuggets: Breaded and fried, often containing high amounts of unhealthy fats.
3. Tacos and Burritos: Particularly those with ground beef, cheese, sour cream, and guacamole. Again, if you choose to eat these foods, choose one high calorie fat ingredient you prefer most and leave out the others.

Pastries and Desserts

1. Doughnuts: Fried and often covered in sugary coatings or filled with creams.
2. Pastries: Croissants, danishes, and other pastries are often made with large amounts of butter or shortening.
3. Cheesecakes: High in fat due to cream cheese and often topped with sugary glazes.

Sauces and Dressings

1. Cream-Based Sauces: Alfredo, béchamel, and other cream-based

sauces are typically high in butter and cream.

2. Salad Dressings: Especially creamy dressings like ranch, Caesar, and blue cheese, which often contain oils, mayonnaise, or buttermilk.

3. Gravy: Often made with meat drippings and butter or cream.

Cheese-Laden Dishes

1. Pizza: Especially with extra cheese or meat toppings.

2. Macaroni and Cheese: Typically made with large amounts of cheese and often with butter or cream.

3. Cheese-Stuffed Items: Mozzarella sticks, jalapeno poppers, and enchiladas.

Meat Dishes

1. Steaks and Ribs: Particularly those with visible marbling of fat or served with butter or creamy sauces.

2. Pork Belly and Bacon: High in saturated fats and often cooked in additional fats.

3. Sausages and Meatballs: Often contain high amounts of fat, particularly saturated fats.

4. Chicken, Tuna and Egg Salads: Made with large amounts of mayonnaise.

Side Dishes

1. Mashed Potatoes: Typically made with butter, cream, or cheese.

2. Loaded Baked Potatoes: Topped with butter, sour cream, cheese, and bacon.

3. Refried Beans: Cooked with lard or oils and topped with cheese.

4. Coleslaw: Often made with mayonnaise-based dressings.

Breads and Spreads

1. Garlic Bread: Usually made with butter or margarine.
2. Corn Bread: Often made with butter and sugar.
3. Buttered Rolls: Bread rolls served with butter or brushed with oil.

Certain Ethnic Specialty Foods

1. Mexican Dishes: Enchiladas, Chile Rellenos, Chimichangas which are often cheese-laden and/or deep fried.
2. Chinese Dishes: Sweet and Sour or Orange dishes, deep-fried and coated in sugary, fatty sauces.
3. Italian Pasta Dishes: Cream-based pastas like fettuccine alfredo or carbonara.
4. Indian Curries: Often made with ghee (clarified butter) or heavy cream.

When dining out, it's helpful to be aware of these high-fat items and consider opting for grilled, steamed, or baked alternatives. Requesting sauces and dressings on the side and choosing dishes with more vegetables can also help reduce fat and calorie intake. Making small modifications, such as asking for leaner cuts of meat or whole-grain options, can contribute significantly to making healthier dining choices and keeping the calories in line with your weight and heath goals.

5

Think Mediterranean Diet and You'll Cover the Bases for Healthy Eating

What exactly is the "Mediterranean Diet"? For the past 7 years the Mediterranean Diet has earned the number one spot in U.S. News & World Report's annual Best Diets list as the best diet overall to follow. It's actually not just a diet - it's a way of life. Living a Mediterranean lifestyle involves more than just following a specific diet; it's about embracing a holistic approach to health and well-being. Here are the key components:

1. **Healthy Eating:** Focus on consuming fresh, whole foods rich in nutrients. The Mediterranean diet is a heavily plant-based way of eating and emphasizes lots of vegetables and fruits, whole grains, legumes, nuts, and healthy fats like olive oil. Fish and seafood are preferred over red meat, and dairy is consumed in moderation.

2. **Physical Activity:** Regular physical activity is a cornerstone. This includes walking, cycling, swimming, and other forms of moderate exercise. Staying active helps maintain a healthy body and mind.

3. **Social Connections:** Strong social ties are vital. Meals are often

26

shared with family and friends, fostering a sense of community and belonging. This social interaction is linked to increased happiness and better mental health.

4. **Moderation:** Eating in moderation is key. Portion control and mindful eating help maintain a balanced diet without overindulgence.

5. **Relaxation and Stress Management:** Prioritizing relaxation and managing stress are crucial. This can include taking time for leisure activities, enjoying nature, and practicing mindfulness or meditation.

6. **Adequate Sleep:** Getting enough sleep is essential for overall health. Aim for 7-9 hours of quality sleep each night to support physical and mental well-being.

7. **Enjoyment of Life:** Embrace a positive outlook and find joy in everyday activities. Happiness and contentment are integral to the Mediterranean way of life.

Including all of the above can lead to a long and healthy life full of contentment and well being. Give it a try!

6

Calories Count and Estimating is Easy

Understanding and managing calorie intake is a crucial aspect of maintaining a healthy diet and achieving your weight and health goals. This chapter provides information on how to determine your total daily calorie budget and why it's important to know your number, practical tips on estimating calorie counts, using available nutritional information, and making lower-calorie swaps that won't compromise on taste.

Know Your Calorie Budget

Knowing your daily caloric needs is crucial in managing weight and is based on your health goals. If your goal is to maintain your weight, the calories you eat need to balance very closely with the amount of calories you burn each day. If you are trying to lose weight, you will need to eat significantly fewer calories than you burn. On the other hand, if you eat more calories than you burn, the excess calories will be stored as fat, and the type of calories doesn't matter - whether it's too much protein, too many carbs, or too much fat. Too many calories above your daily calorie budget equals weight gain.

How to Determine Your Personal Daily Calorie Budget

The best way to figure out how many calories you burn each day is to either use online calculators or consult with a dietitian to find out what's appropriate for you.

Recruit an RDN: The ideal resource to use to determine your personal calorie budget would be a Registered Dietitian Nutritionist who has access to equipment and professional calculators specifically designed to accurately determine a person's calorie expenditure. You can search for registered dietitians in your area online and you should find multiple options. This may not always be practical so the next best option would be to try one of the online calorie calculators.

Use an Online Calculator: Here are some reliable online calorie calculators that can help you determine your daily calorie budget based on your individual needs:

1. Eat This Much Calorie Calculator: This tool can calculate your calorie and macronutrient targets and can help set realistic weight goals.
2. Mayo Clinic Calorie Calculator: One of the more respected resources in the field of medicine, this calculator gives you a very good estimate of the number of calories your body expends daily using your current age, height, weight and activity level. It also gives you options should your activity levels change.
3. Calculator.net: This calculator estimates the number of calories your body requires daily and gives foal intake ranges for slow to fast weight loss.

Quick and Easy Estimate: As a Registered Dietitian Nutritionist myself, I am often asked to provide a general calorie budget estimation as a quick and simple guideline for someone who is in need of an estimate and does not have time to do a regular consultation. In those cases here is what I typically recommend: In a pinch, women can safely aim for a daily calorie budget of about 1500-1600 calories, unless they are highly active in sports or exercise, in which case I would then recommend 1800-2000 calories. Men can aim for a daily calorie budget of about 2000-2200 calories, unless they are highly active, in which case I would recommend 2600-2800 calories.

NOTE: These ranges are intended to be used in general and on occasion, however it is ideal to obtain a more accurate calorie budget by using a calorie estimator or consulting with a Registered Dietitian Nutritionist.

Tips on Estimating Calorie Content of Foods

Understanding your daily caloric needs and staying within your calorie budget is always important to consider when dining out. However, it can be challenging to know exactly how many calories you are actually consuming when you eat, especially if nutritional information isn't readily available. Here are some tips to help you successfully manage your calorie intake with your food choices:

1. **Look for Posted Calorie Information:** Many restaurants, especially chains, now post calorie counts on their menus. Use this information to help make decisions that fit within your calorie budget.

2. **Use Apps and Online Tools:** There are many smartphone apps and online databases that provide calorie counts for common restaurant dishes. Use these tools to get a good estimate of your meal's calorie content. Some of my favorite calorie tracking apps are MyNetDiary, Myfitnesspal, and Lose It, although there may be others that are more appealing to each individual. The best app to use is the one you will use frequently! Make sure the app you

choose can monitor your macros, fiber, sodium, added sugars, and many other important nutrients, and you'll find that many popular restaurants have the calorie and nutritional content of their menu items included in those apps. It can also help to find similar dishes at other restaurants. Example: a meal you are eating is similar to other items in the apps and ranges from 160 to 340 calories. Take the average (let's say 250 calories) and use that as your estimate. It won't be exact, but it's a fair estimate. One additional note: it's always a good idea to air on the side of caution and round up a bit to account for any hidden calories coming from extra butter or oil.

3. **Balance Out Your Total Meal:** If you wish to indulge in a higher-calorie appetizer or dessert, adjust your main course to be lighter. Balance high-calorie items with lower-calorie sides or beverages.

4. **Familiarize Yourself with Portions:** Learn what standard portion sizes look like. For example, a healthy serving of meat is roughly the size of a deck of cards, and a serving of rice or pasta is about the size of a tennis ball. Vegetables and fruits are unlimited when it comes to portions! As long as they are steamed or without creams or sugary sauces, eat as many as you'd like. They are highly nutritious, typically low calorie, and they create lots of volume which can fill you up quickly.

5. **Break Down the Ingredients:** If you know the main ingredients in a dish, estimate the calorie content of each component. For example, a grilled chicken breast is around 200 calories, while a side of steamed vegetables is usually between 50-100 calories without the butter, and a cup of pasta or rice is typically 200 calories a handful.

6. **Estimate When Necessary:** If calorie information isn't available, estimate based on similar items you know or search online for food establishments that provide nutritional information for the foods you are considering eating. If you can find the calorie content of

similar dishes from other places or from home-cooked meals, use that information as a benchmark.

Using Available Nutritional Information

Many restaurants, especially larger chains, provide nutritional information for their menu items. Here's how to make the most of it:

1. **Check Before You Go**: Look up nutritional information on the restaurant's website before you visit. This can help you make informed choices ahead of time. If you don't see calories or other nutrition information posted, search another restaurant that you are familiar with that may offer similar menu items.
2. **Ask for Nutritional Information:** If the information isn't readily available, ask your server. Many restaurants have nutritional brochures or can provide information upon request.
3. **Focus on Key Nutrients:** Pay attention to calories posted, but also consider other important factors like fat, sugar, and sodium content. A meal low in calories but high in sodium, saturated fats, or sugar may not be the healthiest choice.

Making Lower-Calorie Swaps Without Sacrificing Taste

You don't have to sacrifice taste to enjoy lower-calorie meals. Here are some strategies to make delicious, healthier choices:

1. **Choose Grilled Over Fried**: Opt for grilled, baked, roasted, or steamed dishes instead of fried ones. Grilled foods often have a similar taste but significantly fewer calories.
2. **Request Sauces and Dressings on the Side**: Sauces and dressings add flavor and a desirable mouth feel, but they also can add a lot of hidden calories. Since the sauces or dressings typically create the uniqueness of the meal, it's completely understandable why you

would want to include those flavors in your meal, and you should! Just ask for them on the side and use them sparingly to control how much you consume.

3. **Opt for Clear Soups Over Creamy Ones:** Clear, broth-based soups typically have fewer calories than creamy soups, which are often made with high-fat ingredients. Look for ones with lots of vegetables added instead of meats and cheeses.

4. **Customize Your Order:** Don't be afraid to ask for modifications. Request less cheese, no mayo, or extra vegetables to reduce calorie content and make your meal more nutritious without sacrificing flavor. If you see an ingredient listed in the dish on the menu, you most likely can modify it or leave it out.

5. **Know exactly what's in the meal you are choosing:** Sometimes the description of a menu item isn't clear, often containing only a few descriptive words of what it contains. If you are not sure what ingredients are included or how it is prepared, ask the staff at the place where you are dining. Some ingredients are often left off the menu description, such as butter or wine, and these hidden ingredients can hike up the total calories even in small amounts.

6. **Choose Lean Proteins:** Select lean protein sources such as chicken breast, turkey, fish, or plant-based proteins over higher-fat options like beef or pork. You'll still get equivalent amounts of protein but with significantly less calories.

7. **Drink Water or Unsweetened Beverages:** Sugary drinks can add a lot of extra calories. Opt for water, sparkling water, or unsweetened tea instead of sugar sweetened sodas or juices which will help you stay hydrated without the added calories. **One rule of thumb we dietitians stand by - don't drink your calories.**

By learning how to estimate calorie counts, using available nutritional information, and making strategic lower-calorie swaps, you can enjoy dining out while staying on track with your health and weight manage-ment goals. In the next chapter, we will conclude our guide with some additional tips and a summary of the key points covered, helping you dine out with confidence and maintain your health goals. No matter what, don't go into your meal blind. Take the few minutes it might require to research a little about what you are about to eat. It can make a huge difference in achieving your goals to maintain, lose, or even gain weight and ultimately achieve the healthy body you desire.

7

Additional Tips for Keeping Meals Healthy and Portion Controlled

As we have seen so far, dining out can be a very enjoyable and satisfying experience, but it often comes with challenges such as controlling calorie intake, resisting temptations, and managing portion sizes. This chapter provides some additional and very practical tips to help you keep your meals healthy and portion-controlled, ensuring you stay on track with your health and weight management goals.

Doggie Bag a Portion of Your Meal BEFORE You Start Eating It

One effective way to manage portion sizes and reduce calorie intake is to ask for a to-go box as soon as your meal is served. Portion off a part of it into the to-go container. Use the MyPlate guidelines to visualize appropriate portion sizes, serve yourself a healthy MyPlate meal, and then pack up and save the rest for another meal.

Share Plates

Sharing dishes with your dining companions is a great strategy to enjoy a variety of foods while keeping portions in check:

1. **Order for Sharing:** Choose a few dishes that everyone at the table can share. This way, you can taste different foods without overindulging. And if there are just two of you, choose an appetizer or salad to share, then choose a main dish that works to share for both of you.
2. **Balance Choices:** Include a mix of healthy options such as salads, vegetable sides, and lean proteins along with any small indulgence you may wish to enjoy and share such as a higher calorie appetizer or decadent dessert.

Find Substitutions for Higher Calorie Ingredients

Many restaurants are willing to accommodate requests for healthier ingredient substitutions. Here are some ideas:

1. **Healthier Cooking Methods:** Request your food to be grilled, steamed, or baked instead of fried or sauteed.
2. **Swap Out Ingredients:** Substitute higher-calorie ingredients with healthier options, such as replacing creamy dressings with vinai-grettes, egg whites instead of whole eggs, grilled chicken breast burger instead of hamburger, or whole grain bread instead of white bread.
3. **Light on the Sauces:** Ask for sauces and dressings on the side so you can control how much you use, and try subbing plain ketchup or mustard for mayo or oil-based condiments. The calorie savings definitely add up.

Read Menus and Make Your Meal Decisions Before Going to the Restaurant

Planning ahead can help you make healthier choices and avoid impulsive decisions:

1. **Decide Before You Dine:** Look up the restaurant's menu online before you go and decide what you will order. This helps you stick to your health goals.
2. **Identify Healthy Options:** Look for meals that are labeled as healthy, low-calorie, or heart-healthy, and plan to order those.

Look Over the Menu and Find Alternate, Healthier Sides to Add to Your Meal

Many meals come with sides that can be high in calories, such as fries, mashed potatoes, or creamy coleslaw, but you don't have to settle for what is offered with your meal choice. Here's how to choose better alternatives:

1. **Vegetable Sides**: Opt for vegetable sides like steamed broccoli or spinach, side salads, grilled vegetables, or baked potato (hold the "loaded"), instead of fries or mashed potatoes. If you see a vegetable that interests you but is prepared with high fat ingredients like oil, butter, or cream, ask if it can be prepared steamed only.
2. **Whole Grains**: Choose sides like brown rice, quinoa, or whole wheat pasta over white rice or refined grains.
3. **Fruit:** Adding a side of fresh fruit can be a healthy and refreshing alternative to heavier sides.

Share Desserts, or Take One or Two Bites and Take the Rest Home

Desserts can be a significant source of extra calories, but you don't have to skip them entirely:

1. **Share Desserts:** Split a dessert with your dining companions to enjoy a few bites without consuming the whole portion.

2. **Mindful Tasting:** Take one or two bites to satisfy your sweet tooth, then ask for the rest to be boxed up to enjoy later.

3. **Focus on Fruits:** Desserts that include fresh fruits such as berries or melon, as well as fruit sorbets are a great way to satisfy a sweet tooth and pack a nutritional punch at the same time.

Choose Meals from the Kids' Menu or the Appetizer Section for Your Main Meal

Smaller portions from the kids' menu or appetizer section can be a smart way to manage portion sizes and calorie intake:

1. **Kid-Sized Portions:** Kids' meals often come in smaller portions, which can be just the right amount of food. Pair with a side salad or vegetable dish to create a healthy, balanced meal.

2. **Appetizer Options:** Appetizers are typically smaller than main courses so again, pair with a side salad, soup, or vegetable dish to create a healthy, balanced meal.

3. **Balanced Pairing:** Look for soup and salad, soup and sandwich, or salad and sandwich combos. They typically include smaller portions of each and can create a healthier, more balanced meal.

Other techniques to help you manage your calories and ensure you have a healthy meal.

1. **Eat a small portion of a healthy, lower calorie food before you head out.** Sometimes we do not have a say in where we are going, and we know in advance that we are going to be eating at a high calorie, indulgent restaurant. In this case, one very successful strategy to help you avoid overindulging is to eat something small and healthy just before heading out to the restaurant. Some suggestions are: have a hefty serving of fruit; make a small, healthy shake with

protein and fruit in it; eat a nutrition bar; have a few handfuls of veggies and hummus; enjoy a serving of yogurt or cottage cheese along with a little bit of fruit; or even something like a handful of pretzels and grapes could stave off the hangries and help with better self control when ordering off the menu.

2. **Always include at least one vegetable or fruit to your meal**. Even the leanest proteins and healthiest whole grain carbs won't provide optimal nutrition if there are no vegetables or fruits included with the meal.

3. **Think MyPlate every time you eat** to ensure you have all of its main components - healthy starches/carbs, lean proteins, and plenty of vegetables and/or fruits to complete the nutritional balance of your meal. Your body will thank you!

8

Conclusion

No matter what, DON'T STRESS! It's just food, and it's not about getting all of these tips perfect every time. It's about being willing to make changes, no matter how small, that eventually will add up to great health benefits as you continue to add in more and more. By incorporating even just one or two of these tips, you can begin to enjoy dining out while making your meals healthier and closer to your calorie budget, and learn to acquire a new found taste for "healthy". Bon appetit!

I do have one special request. If you found this book helpful, please take a moment to leave a favorable review for my book on Amazon. My goal is to reach as many people as possible around the world with these tips on eating healthier so they, too, can reap some amazing health benefits, and your reviews can make that happen! Thank you for reading my book.

9

Resources

MyPlate | U.S. Department of Agriculture. (n.d.). https://www.myplate.gov/

U.S. News Reveals the 2024 Best Diets: Mediterranean diet tops list for seventh consecutive year. (2024). *U.S. News & World Report.* https://www.usnews.com/info/blogs/press-room/articles/2024-01-03/u-s-news-reveals-the-2024-best-diets

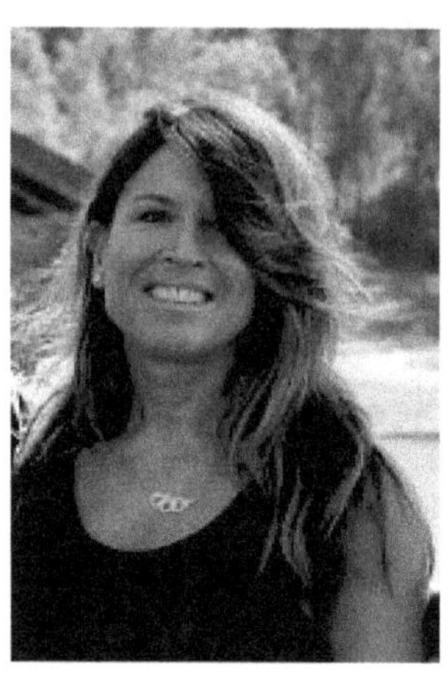

About the Author

I was born and raised in NY and moved to CA in 1987 to pursue art and interior design. I stumbled into the bodybuilding world in 1988 and became obsessed with exercise and nutrition and how both can contribute to a beautifully sculpted, healthy body - inside and out. I am fascinated by the workings of the human body and how our diet and lifestyle affect every single cell, positively or negatively. I left my art and design career behind and pursued what has now become my life's passion - Health & Wellness. I have been a Registered Dietitian Nutritionist since 2000 and have helped hundreds of people of all ages, ethnicities, and socioeconomic backgrounds lose weight, get healthier, and become proactive in taking control of their own health. And I practice what I preach. In other words - *I walk the talk.* I have benefited greatly and I want to share what I have learned so that others can experience the same vitality and zest for life. I have the same energy now as I had in my 30's, and as of the time I am writing this book, I am in my 60's.

I started my own healthy lifestyle program in 2019 called **h.e.a.r.t.s.**

Lifestyle Program where I teach weekly classes to seniors, and also provide private consultations to all ages for weight loss, sports nutrition and athletic performance, and general health and wellness.

My hopes in writing this book, along with many more to come, are to reach a many people as possible around the world with the coaching, knowledge, and motivation to become their healthiest they can be, knowing it is possible to get healthier at any age, and be able to truly enjoy a full life of healthy longevity.

If anyone would like to contact me and learn more about what I do, my email address is: dmotise@heartslifestyle.com.

You can connect with me on:

🌐 https://heartslifestyle.com

f https://www.facebook.com/dianemotise22?mibextid=kFxxJD

🔗 https://www.instagram.com/h.e.a.r.t.s.lifestyle